Hair Care Like A Pro

Professional Hair Care Tips on Getting Shinier, Prettier, Healthier Hair, How to Grow Long Hair, & How to Choose the Right Products for Your Hair Type

Evelyn R. Scott
Copyright© 2014 by Evelyn R. Scott

Hair Care Like A Pro

Publisher: Enlightened Publishing

ISBN-13: 978-1500836467

ISBN-10: 150083646X

Disclaimer

The Publisher has strived to be as accurate and complete as possible in the creation of this book. While all attempts have been made to verify information provided in this publication, the Publisher assumes no responsibility for errors, omissions, or contrary interpretation of the subject matter herein. Any perceived slights of specific persons, peoples, or organizations are unintentional.

This book is not intended for use as a source of legal, business, accounting or financial advice. All readers are advised to seek services of competent professionals in the legal, business, accounting, and finance fields.

The information in this book is not intended or implied to be a substitute for professional medical advice, diagnosis or treatment. All content contained in this book is for general information purposes only. Always consult your healthcare provider before carrying on any health program.

Table of Contents

Introduction

In today's modern world, we typically think of our hair as an accessory. It can enhance our beauty to make us more glamorous, more serious, cutting edge, whimsical or youthful. There are a lot of stereotypes that revolve around hairstyles and even colors. Blondes are less intelligent, but tend to have more fun, right? Well, we all know that's not necessarily the case.

Biologically, our hair serves the purpose of protecting our skin against the elements – that's truly why it's there. But because we have evolved and created many ways to protect ourselves over the centuries, hair tends to simply be an adornment.

It seems that some people can be obsessed with the style of their hair. If it's short they want it longer. If it's long, they consider chopping it off. Blondes eye brunette locks and wonder if they'd look better in darker hair.

And those with naturally curly hair covet pin-straight hair that doesn't even have the slightest wave to it.

While we go about changing our hair to the style we desire, it's important to first understand what our hair is like at its foundation. If it's naturally oily or dry, thick or thin, coarse or fine and whether or not it is predisposed to growing longer, or if it will simply look thin and wispy if it grows beyond our shoulders.

There are certainly ways to synthetically enhance your natural hair, but learning to work with what you've got – and learning to like it, too – will go a long way in easing frustration about your hair as you try to drastically alter it.

That being sad, this guide sets out to help you define you natural hair and its built-in strengths and weaknesses. Knowing that, we discuss the proper routine products you should be using and how to create more natural versions that don't have the typical chemicals that will strip the outer layer of your hair and make it look dull. Plus you'll learn tips for getting your hair to grow longer and more luxuriously as well as diet tips that can drastically improve the appearance of your hair and habits of women whose hair always looks great.

For those who still want to alter their hair, this guide covers the safest ways to do that for your personal hair type. Trying to veer too far away from what you've naturally got is a recipe for disaster. So read on to learn more about appreciating your own hair type and making it looks the best that it can – no matter what your age.

Chapter 1: What's Your Hair Type?

The natural state of your hair can be characterized in three main ways: moisture, texture and thickness. Your hair may defined by one of each of these categories. For example, you might have dry, wavy, thick hair. Or maybe you've got oily, straight, fine hair. There are a lot of ways hair can be characterized – and a variety of ways to manage it – but let's define each to help you determine what kind of hair you have.

Moisture Types

Dry hair

Like the rest of your skin, your scalp contains sebaceous glands that secrete a type of oil called sebum. This oil is important for the scalp and hair because it provides essential moisturizing qualities and protects the scalp from environmental elements.

Similar to the way it affects the skin on your face, a lack of sufficient sebum production will make your hair drier. If your hair is not properly hydrated with sebum, it can feel straw-like, break easily, develop split ends and have an overall dull appearance.

This lack of sebum can simply be genetic, but it is also affected by environmental hazards (like too much sun or hair-altering chemicals), low-quality or the wrong formula of hair-care products or even your diet.

Oily hair

Conversely, oily hair typically has an overproduction of sebum that gives hair a greasy look. Too much sebum can also be genetic or caused by factors like stress and bad diet, as well as overuse of chemicals or the wrong hair-care products. Even when it's been recently washed, oily hair can look dirty, heavy and appear to stick to the scalp. Sweating excessively and eating the wrong foods can also cause hair to appear greasy. However, washing oily hair too frequently will strip the outer layer – or cuticle – which is what makes the hair look shiny. So people with truly oily often have dried out ends.

Normal or combination hair

The majority of people have characteristics of both oily and dry hair. While their scalp may be oily, the ends may be frayed. People with healthy, normal hair have strands that have fluid-like movement, are shiny and do not split at the ends.

To determine your hair moisture type, wash your hair and wait a day. The next day, take a piece of tissue paper and blot (but don't rub) the top of your head and the sides of your head behind your ears. If the tissue does not pick up any oil, you have oilier hair. If it is laden with oil, you have oily hair. If the tissue is mostly dry and your hair has a shine to it, you're one of the lucky ones who have normal, healthy hair.

Your hair's ability to absorb moisture will also play a role in how your hair looks. The outer "cuticle" of your hair's structure may be tight or loose, which will determine how much moisture goes in and out of your hair. A cuticle that is very compact is hard to process and style, while very porous hair is the opposite and susceptible to being over-processed or damaged very easily when coloring or styling. If your hair feels straw-like when dry, it is probably compact. If it has a rubbery feel when wet, it's likely to be very porous.

Is your hair very elastic? This is an important element of hair health, as well. When it's dry, healthy hair will stretch about 20 percent from its natural shape. When it's wet, it can stretch up to 50 percent. To test your hair's elasticity, take four strands of your wet hair from different areas of your head. If you pull on the hair and it stretches without breaking, it's it good shape. If it breaks easily, it's lacking in elasticity, which could make it more likely to suffer split ends and break when styling.

Texture Types

Straight hair

The texture of your hair begins with genetics and at the hair follicle – the opening the hair grows out of your scalp. The follicles can be different shapes, from flat to round to oval. People with straight hair have follicles that are circular, and when the hair grows, it does not twist as much as other hair types. This hair follicle shape can change with fluctuating hormones or medication use, so some people who originally had pin-straight hair may see more of a slight wave to their hair. Those with straight hair may experience more oily moisture levels because the sebum can more easily travel down straight hair and weigh it down.

Wavy

Typically, people with wavy hair have oval-shaped hair follicles and more twists when the hair grows than people with straight hair. This usually results in an "S" shaped wave to the hair. Wavy-hair types may be more affected by humidity in the air, which the hair absorbs and causes it to curl more or even look frizzy.

Curly

At the base of every hair follicle is what's called a hair bulb. For those with curlier hair, this bulb has a hooked shaped that makes hair grow at an angle. Curly-haired people also have a flatter, more oval-shaped hair follicle – resulting in curlier strands that have a "Z" shape to them as they grow. Also, it may have more protein elements in that make it curlier.

The intensity of the curl can vary from very loose to tight corkscrew curls to kinky, coily hair, often found among African hair.

Curly hair tends to be drier than straight hair because the sebum gets trapped closer to the skin. In high humidity, curly hair will absorb more moisture and cause it to go straighter – which typically just looks frizzy.

Thickness Types

Thick or thin hair

Determining if your hair is thick or thin is basically a genetic difference of how many hair follicles you have. The more hair follicles and strands of hair you have growing out of them the thicker your hair is. Someone with medium-thick hair has about 2,200 hair follicles per square inch on their scalp – blondes typically have the most hairs-per-inch, while redheads have the fewest.

Fine or coarse hair

Although most people associate fine hair with thin hair, the truth is that you can actually have thick and fine hair, too. If you have fine hair, it simply means that the diameter of each individual strand is small. Coarse hair has a larger diameter per strand, making it stronger than fine hair. So you can certainly have a lot of very small strands or fewer very big strands. One easy way to determine if you have fine hair is to pull it back into a ponytail. Is it a voluminous or a skinny ponytail? Fine hair will look thinner once it's in a ponytail.

Fine hair tends to be more fragile and can break more easily and appear oilier. Coarse hair, on the other hand, tends to appear drier. One way to tell is to time how long it takes for your hair to dry naturally. Fine hair will be dry in less than an hour, whereas coarse hair takes more than an hour to dry without the help of a blow drier. Also, once dry, course hair will look duller without the help of styling products.

Coarse hair may be more difficult to curl with heating tools and it may also take more time to alter with chemicals, whereas fine hair adapts more quickly – but is also subject to more damage. Interestingly, hair thickness is not defined by ethnic background. All races have been found to have fine or coarse hair thicknesses.

How your hair changes with age

It's obvious that our hair changes through our lifetime. Many of us started out with very light blonde, thin hair that grew thicker and darker over the childhood years. Human hair typically starts thinner at birth, then grows thicker through early adulthood, and once again thins with age.

While most people are focused on the pigment of their hair as the age – and whether it will lose pigment and turn gray – the truth is that your hair moisture levels, texture and thickness can change with age as well.

Individual hairs can continue growing on your head for four or five years before they go through the natural hair growth cycle and eventually fall out. The only truly living part of your hair is at the hair follicle. The main change in the hair follicle is that, with age, it will produce fewer or thinner hair strands. Scientists don't know exactly why these changes happen, but in fact, the follicles do appear to change every five to seven years, but they have some theories.

For women, hormonal changes after about age 40 can alter the thickness of the hair and even result in some level of hair loss – although it is usually minor. Emotional or physical stress can make this hair loss worse. There are some medications and treatments that can slow down this hair loss process. You may begin to notice that your hair dries or curls faster when you use a blow drier or curling iron. Pay attention to how your hair is behaving so that you don't damage it by over-using heating tools.

Women may also find that the moisture levels of their hair changes with time – particularly that their hair becomes drier. As with other cell function within the body, the hair follicle cells begin to work more slowly and the production of sebum is reduced. This will eventually cause a noticeable difference in how oily or dry the hair is. It is believed that your sebum production is reduced by 10 percent for every decade you live.

One of the most common ways women deal with aging hair is by finding a cut that works well with their changing hair. Going shorter may make thin hair look fuller, although there's no rule about how long or short your hair should be at a certain age. Also, experimenting with different products geared toward making hair shinier, thicker or more under control can also help. Instead of choosing chemicals, many natural products will help the hair retain moisture and elasticity as it ages.

If it seems like your favorite products are no longer "working" it may be due to the fact that your hair is changing from a more oily texture to a drier texture. Consider switching up your shampoo, conditioner, and styling products as your hair is changing.

There are many things you can do to slow down the effects of aging hair, including improving your diet with vitamins A, B and E and nutrients that are believed to boost hair density; regular cuts and conditioning treatments; and lessening the use of heated styling tools.

There's not a lot you can do for hair that is losing its pigmentation and turning gray, but if you opt to color it, go for an all-over permanent color rather than trying to fix only certain areas. When your hair starts to go gray, its texture changes as well – typically becoming more coarse and wiry. It's best to have a professional alter the color than trying to do it at home by yourself.

Chapter 2: Maintenance for Your Hair Type

You may know some friends who can go several days without washing their hair, but if you don't wash every day, you end up with a head full of oily-looking hair. Because everyone's hair is different, washing and conditioning needs vary from person to person. In addition to your hair type, you may have other needs as well, such as scalp conditions like dandruff. Here are some guidelines for good, regular hair-care routines.

Washing Your Hair

Because most shampoos contain a mixture of detergents, foaming agents, fragrances and other elements, using them too frequently will strip your hair of its natural oils, also known as sebum. While some people naturally have more sebum than others, they can wash their hair more frequently without stripping their hair too much.

Shampoos made specifically for oily hair may be called "claifying," while shampoos for dry hair may be labeled as "moisturizing." Be sure to pick the right formula for your hair type. An oily-hair shampoo will contain more cleansing agents to help keep excess sebum under control. But if you have dry hair, you don't want to eliminate too much of your hair's natural oils.

How often you wash your hair will be determined on your type of hair as well. If you have combination hair, you may want to wash your hair every other day, focusing on the shampooing the scalp and not lathering up the ends. People with thicker and wavy or curly hair can typically go longer between washes – perhaps twice a week. This is because the sebum doesn't travel as easily into thick hair that has a natural curl to it.

However, people with straight, fine hair may find that their sebum production affects their hair in as little as a day, and they feel they need to wash every day. If this is the case, using a gentle and/or natural shampoo is the best strategy. Also, if you have oily hair, you may want to wash it after exercising or other activities that cause you to sweat. A hairstylist can offer the best direction on how often to wash your hair and what types of products to select.

Follow these steps when washing your hair:

- Soak your hair completely under warm running water for about a minute. Don't use water that is too hot.

- Squirt about a quarter-size amount of shampoo in your hand and rub your palms together to spread the shampoo out.

- Start by massaging the shampoo into your scalp, where there is the most excess oil and dirt build-up.

- If your hair is oily, avoid scrubbing your scalp too much, as this can activate your hair follicles into producing more sebum. Conversely, if you have dry hair, massage the scalp a little longer.

- To resist tangles, use your finger tips to massage the shampoo into your hair.

- Completely rinse your hair with warm water until there are no soap bubbles remaining.

- Repeat the cleaning process if needed. If your hair is oily, repeat the lathering process and leave the shampoo on your hair for about five minutes to really cleanse hair fully.

- Some experts believe that a finishing rinse of cold water will help to keep excess sebum production at bay.

- You can follow up with conditioner, which we'll describe next.

Conditioning Your Hair

Moisturizing your hair can be tricky, because if you use too much, it can cause your hair to look limp. But if you don't use enough, your hair may be difficult to comb or brush and look overly dry. The best way to combat this is to choose a conditioner that is right for your hair's natural moisture type (oily, combination or dry) and is appropriate for the texture of your hair (fine, coarse, thin or thick). Reading the labels may take a few extra minutes, but you'll be glad that you did.

There are also a variety of conditioning types – rinse out, deep conditioning and leave-in. A rinse-out condition is good for everyday or every-other-day use. If you wash your hair often, you may want to only condition the ends and stay away from the scalp so as to avoid build up on conditioner that can make any hair type look flat.

A deep conditioner can be used once or twice a week and can be alternated with a rinse-out conditioner. You'll want to follow the directions on the label, as some deep conditioners would in as little as a few minutes, but others must be leave on for up to 15 minutes. These are particularly useful for people with dry hair or tresses that have been damaged by environmental elements, exposure to the sun or excessive chemicals, such as hair coloring and perms. Typically, when using a deep conditioner, you'll rinse it out after the appropriate amount of time has elapsed.

A leave-in conditioner is one that you don't need to rinse out, therefore they are usually lighter formulas that can help eliminate tangles and give your hair a little extra shine and manageability. Be sure to use the leave-in on the ends of your hair rather than at the roots, where it can build up. These can be used in addition to a rinse-out conditioner or on their own, depending on how much moisture your hair needs.

When conditioning your hair, keep these tips in mind:

- After shampooing, you may need to blot your hair dry a little bit before applying the conditioner. You can also do this by very gently squeezing the excess water from your hair with your hands.

- Use a dime- to quarter-size amount of conditioner in your hand, depending on the length of your hair, but do not use more than a quarter-size.

- Focus on applying the conditioner to the length of your hair, but if you've had a particularly dry or flaky scalp, condition the scalp as well.

- You may use a wide-tooth comb to work the conditioner through your hair, but be especially careful because hair is most sensitive when it is wet.

- Pay extra attention to coating the ends of your hair with conditioner.

- When you rinse your hair, run your fingers through it to help the water rinse away all the residual conditioner. You need to fully rinse it out so that any potentially remaining conditioner does not weigh your hair down once it has dried.

Drying Your Hair

How you dry your hair is nearly as important as how you wash and condition it. The most important thing to remember about drying your hair is that you should not rub it between your hands with a towel. When your hair is wet, it is at its most vulnerable and can very easily break or tangle. Instead, simply blot your hair dry by placing the towel over your head and pressing your hands against the towel. Then, roll it into a turban and let it remain rolled up for 10 minutes or so before carefully unwrapping it.

Use a wide-tooth comb to remove the tangles. Work from the ends of the hair up in short strokes up to the top of the head. Running a comb through very tangled hair from the scalp to the ends will likely snap the hair along the way. Another good rule of thumb is to allow it to air dry as often as possible without the help of heating tools like a blow drier.

Haircuts and Trims

As a part of your regular hair maintenance, getting frequent cuts or trims to your hair will ensure that it stays healthy-looking. No matter what products say, once your ends have frayed into split ends, there's no way to fix them. They need to be cut off. If you do not cut them, split ends will continue to travel up the length of the strand of hair, which will eventually force you to cut off more hair to achieve healthier-looking hair.

Your hair grows about a half an inch a month, so if you want to maintain your style, regardless of the length of your hair, it's best to get a cut every four to five weeks, especially if you have a short style. If you're trying to grow your hair longer, go for a minor trim that takes care of any split ends every six to eight weeks. If you don't notice split ends, you can wait for as long as 10 to 12 weeks to get a cut.

If you have chemically altered hair, such as color, straightening or a perm, you may also want to have your hair trimmed more frequently since these chemicals can damage the hair and cause split ends. If you have a blunt-style cut, you probably will not need to have it cut as often as you will if you have many layers throughout your hair – especially layers that have been cut with a razor.

The Best Hairstyles for Your Hair Type

It's true that your hairstyle will say a lot about you, so perhaps the style you choose should begin with your personality and then work with your hair's texture and color to enhance both equally. Women who are more active and play sports might opt for a short pixie cut, while a girl who likes to hit the town a lot might feel like she needs extra length to pull off a sexier look. On the other hand, business women may choose long or short styles that are reserved and expertly styled so that there are no hairs that are out of place. Conversely, a nature-loving girl may have free-flowing waves and a more creative type will spike, curl, straighten or frizz their hair out as their mood strikes.

If you have oily hair, growing out your bangs may be the best option, since hair that hangs over your forehead can easily collect excess oil. If you do have bangs and your hair is oily, try to wear them parted to the side or gather then up loosely with a pin on the top of your head for a quick fix. Or slide on a wide headband to keep your hair off your forehead. Up-dos, like a French twist or a loose bun, hide oily hair the best, rather than a slicked-back ponytail that will just accentuate the oily area.

If you have dry hair, stay away from short haircuts that can end up looking poofy. Instead, go for shoulder-length hair that has plenty of layers. Getting your hair cut into a bob or a blunt cut can cause dry ends to really stand out, which you don't want to do. If you have dry hair that is naturally curly, let it grow longer. Ask your hairstylist for a haircut that doesn't require daily use of a hair dryer or hot styling tools that will only make your hair drier with regular use.

Those with fine and or thin hair can get away with a dramatic angled bob or even jagged edges that look modern and funky. Using a volumizer at the roots will help give some lift and make these types of styles look their best.

Women with thick hair have a lot of options. They can go short for a low-maintenance look; they can wear a chin-length bob, so long as layers are expertly cut so that the hair doesn't look too wide; or they can opt for longer hair with layers. However, keep in mind that longer hair typically takes more styling and thick and/or coarse hair can take longer to style with heating tools simply because the hair is thicker.

Chapter 3: The Best Products for Your Hair

Going to the beauty supply store to pick out hair products can be a completely over-whelming experience with all of the different brands, types and formulas to choose from. But now that you know what type of hair you have, finding the right products to get your hair to behave properly is the next logical step.

Shampoos for Different Hair Types

Oily hair

Look for naturally nourishing ingredients like ceramides and fatty acids in your sham-poo. For oily hair, it's also important to use a shampoo that has a neutral pH. Plus, products with neutral pH will also help any coloring you've had done to last longer. If you feel like your shampoo isn't keeping the oil from your scalp at bay, it may be because residue from the shampoo is building up on your scalp. Try alternating with a different type from month to month.

Dry hair

Shampoo that is labeled as "smoothing" or "anti-frizz" will help dry-hair types smooth out. Ingredients such as olive oil or avocado oil will coat each strand of hair without making it look greasy and weighed-down.

Aging hair

Look for antioxidants in your shampoo, which will help neutralize free radicals that can cause damage to your hair in a similar way that they damage the skin. Plus, they are also believed to play a role in slowing down hair loss, which becomes more of an issue as women age. Full of vitamins and ingredients like green tea, these shampoos promote follicle health, which in turn helps with hair growth, experts believe.

Conditioners for Different Hair Types

Oily hair

You'll want a light conditioner for oily hair, especially if your roots are oily, yet your ends are dry and brittle. If you suspect that you have a lot of product build-up, you can find some "clarifying" conditioners that leave hair with nothing but shine, thanks to natural ingredients like spring water, botanicals and aloe vera.

Dry hair

Look for conditioners that include the ingredient hyaluronic acid, which is a naturally occurring element in the human body. This acid helps the body to internally retain moisture (like in the knee joints and skin). It can do the same for your hair by filling in rough hair and making it appear smoother because it is able to penetrate deeply within each hair strand.

Natural oils like olive, coconut and nut oils found in moisturizers can give your hair a shot of moisture that looks natural and shiny. If shampooing regularly dries your hair out, you might opt for using a conditioner only on some days. Use a light conditioner that is free of silicones in the ingredient lists. Focus on using the conditioner only on the length of your hair and avoid applying it directly to the scalp when you haven't washed your hair first. Too much conditioner on your scalp will eventually lead to build-up and an over-production of sebum that can make even dry hair look greasy.

Aging hair

Look for shampoos and conditioners that include proteins, especially milk or soy proteins. Because your hair is actually made of proteins as well, these products will help promote healthy locks while protecting it from damaging elements like the sun or pollution. Conditioners that include amino acids, which make up proteins, are believed to help the cells on the hair lay flat, therefore creating shinier, healthier looking hair.

Dry Shampoos

Dry shampoos are a good option if you don't have time to fully wash your hair or if regular shampooing seems to be harsh on your hair or causes it to become too dry. Plus, it's a good option for those who need to soak up the excess oil that may build up in as soon as a day or if you want to retain a salon styling – like a blowout – for a few more days.

Available in spray or powder formulas, dry shampoos are formulated to remove the excess sebum and any dirt or built-up hair styling products that may be weighing your hair down. To use them, you simply brush your hair and spray or sprinkle the product on your scalp and work it through to the rest of your hair. Wait for five to 10 minutes and brush your hair out again to remove any remaining dry shampoo. You may also want to give your hair a gentle rub with a towel before the final brush out if you feel like you have too much product remaining.

Maintenance Products

With combination or dry hair, or hair that's been overly processed with chemicals or heat-based styling tools, it's a good idea to give it a deep conditioning treatment with a mask or oil. Look for ingredients that are known to rehydrate parched hair and provide moisture and shine while preventing future breakage.

Two oils that you can use daily without build-up are argan oil and macadamia oil – both which are fairly new to the hair-care scene, but provide excellent hydration. These amazing oils seem to magically transform fly-aways and frizzy hair into smooth tresses – with judicious use, of course. And they work well on all hair types.

For deep moisturizing effects, try a mask that contains wheat protein to help repair the hair and natural ingredients like fruit oils and shea butter to nourish it deeply and make it shine. Masks that include peptides, sulphur and talc powder will help to absorb sebum from oily hair without stripping the hair bare.

Natural Ingredients and Do-It-Yourself Products

Many hair products that are mass-manufactured today contain a combination of ingredients that are inexpensive for the companies to use and effectively remove oil, dirt and product overload from the hair. These detergent-like ingredients are known as sulfates.

These don't do much harm when we're younger, but as we age, hair becomes more sensitive, thin and prone to breakage, so cutting back on chemicals is more important than ever. Instead, more natural ingredients like antioxidants and proteins can work just as well and even provide extra protection for aging hair. Look for hair-care products that are labeled "sulfate-free," and try to find more natural ingredients like those listed below.

Shampoo

If you're battling oily hair, look for citrus ingredients, like lemon, in the shampoo that can help reduce the oil in your hair. Jojoba oil is another important ingredient for anyone with oily hair or with a scalp issue, like dandruff. Also, adding a few drops of essential oils that are known for their antiseptic qualities to your shampoo can help cut down on oil, like orange or sage essential oils. Aloe vera is believed to boost scalp health, so you can add it directly to your scalp or add a few drops to your daily shampoo.

To make your own shampoo, mix up a cup of water plus a tablespoon of baking soda. After they are mixed well, apply to wet hair and rinse thoroughly.

A cool rinse can help to smooth the hair's cuticle, leaving you with super-shiny locks. Add either white vinegar or lemon to cool water and rinse your hair with it. Or you can also try diluting a few drops of thyme or rosemary oil with a tablespoon of vinegar with mineral water.

For a natural dry shampoo, use corn starch on light-colored hair or cocoa powder for darker shades. The natural powdery substances will help to remove excess oil from your hair.

Conditioners

Conditioners can be expensive, but you can actually find ingredients that will leave your hair smooth and shiny – right in your kitchen. Simply applying eggs, mayonnaise, beer or bananas to your hair for a few minutes will really boost the shine.

You can also make a conditioner at home by mixing up a half of a ripe avocado with about a teaspoon of olive oil and a few drops of lavender essential oil. Simply apply to hair (pay special attention to the ends) and leave on for up to 10 minutes before completely rinsing it out.

For another at-home hair conditioner, combine 1 tablespoon of unflavored gelatine, a cup of water and a teaspoon of cider vinegar to your hair after you wash it with shampoo. Leave it on for five minutes before you rinse it out completely.

Hair Masks

Dry hair types may find that they need an extra boost of moisture, and one good way to achieve that is, once a week, before you wash your hair, use a mask that contains natural ingredients. Here are some good recipes to try at home:

Oil mask

- 2 tablespoons sunflower or castor oil
- 1 tablespoon of macadamia or argan oil
- 5-10 drops lavender oil
- 5 drops clary sage oil

Mix the oils and apply to damp hair and loosely wrap the head with a clear cling wrap. Next take a warm towel (pop it in the dryer for a few minutes) and gently wrap your hair into a turban. Allow your hair to absorb the oil for 15 to 20 minutes before you wash and condition it using your usual products. You can use this oil-based masked every week or two.

Olive oil & honey mask

- 2 tablespoons olive oil
- 2 tablespoons honey
- 1 egg yolk
- 1 tablespoon lemon juice

Warm the oil and honey just until it is a smooth liquid. Add egg yolk and lemon juice and apply the mixture to your hair. Wrap in a warm towel and let it soak for 20 to 30 minutes before following with a shampoo.

Clay mask

- 1 cup powdered clay
- 1 tablespoon vinegar
- Water

Mix the clay and vinegar and then trickle in water until you have the consistency of a thick paste. Apply to hair and let it set for 10 minutes. Wash hair as usual.

You can also combine cocoa butter with coconut water to create a quick hair mask that you apply for about 30 minutes before washing out. It's a super-fragrant hair mask that leaves you hair incredibly shiny.

Chapter 4: Styling Tips for All Hair Types

Beyond washing and conditioning your hair, there are an endless array of styling mousses, gels, serums, brushes, combs and heated tools that promise to make your hair shinier, healthier, more luminescent and all-around sexier. But choosing the wrong product or tool can lead to disastrous effects, like hair that is overloaded with products and looking flat and lifeless. Here are some tips to know when choosing the proper products for your hair type:

Styling Products – Adding Volume to All Hair Types

No matter if your hair is fine and thin or thick and coarse, everyone wants to have voluminous hair that has great movement and bounce to it. When shopping for a volumizer, look for ingredients like starch, which soaks up extra oil, protein that helps your hair's texture, humectants for dry hair and polymers, which help to thicken each strand of hair.

Fine hair can use an extra boost of protein, like wheat extract or soy in a mousse-like volumizer, while thicker hair can also improve with the help of protein in a spray product that helps to tame frizzy hair, plus a soy protein-based spray can also help to lock in moisture. If your hair is dull, look for natural botanical ingredients, like lavender. And anyone with layers or curly hair may find that polymers in certain products will give hair a much-needed lift and better movement.

When using a volumizer product, whether it's a gel, mousse, foam or spray, be sure to follow the instructions on the label and only apply it to the roots of your hair, which is where your hair gets its volume. The best way to do this is to hang your head toward the floor so that your hair is flipped over and you can reach the roots easily.

Adding Extra Shine

There are many serums available that promise to add a head-full of shine in just a few drops. They work by coating the hair's outer cuticle to make it shinier and by adding a layer of protection to stop further damage form the elements. But choosing the proper formula for your hair type is essential. Because sun damage is the number one factor in causing hair to lose its shine, look for a serum that has protective ingredients, like vitamin E, marine extracts and beta-carotene, to add a shield of protection along with some additional shine.

Because oily hair already has enough oil, opt for a light-weight serum that's not too greasy-feeling and will help you to comb out tangles when used on damp hair. A silicone-based serum may be too heavy for thin or oily hair. Dry hair can benefit from a formula that is a bit thicker – perhaps a glaze or pomade instead of an oil – that is left in the hair and acts as a shine booster and a styling aid.

Styling Aids

Mousse

A hair mousse is typically a foam product that can perform a lot of styling wonders for your hair, including adding volume, shine and help to form your particular style – whether it is straight, wavy or curly. It's a great option for thin or fine hair because they are typically lighter than gel or cream styling products. A mousse can work well for either oily hair that needs minimum products or dry hair that needs a bit more moisture.

Read product labels carefully to ensure you choose the right formula for your hair. If your hair is fine, look for words like "volumizing." If your hair is dry, look for "conditioning" and "alcohol-free." Whichever formula you choose, you won't need more than about golf-ball sized mound of foam to cover your hair – less if your hair is short. Some foams also help to protect your hair coloring or even add a bit of temporary color. This can be a big help if your hair is starting to go gray.

Gels

Hair gels have been around for decades, and became particularly popular among men who created those slicked-back styles. However, hair gels have evolved quite a bit since then. You can now find gels in formulas from very lightweight to super-thick. Gels work best on short styles to create fun, spiky looks, but can dry and become flaky on your hair if you work with it too much. It's best to apply when hair is wet, style and then leave it alone. Look for a gel that is tailored to your hair type and the strength of hold that you're looking for.

Hairspray

Like hair gel, hairspray has been around for a long time, but the formulas have multiplied beyond belief. The main purpose of hairspray is to hold your style in place. However, many now offer additional benefits, such as adding shine, conditioning and much more. There are a huge variety of options, and finding the right one may seem overwhelming. To narrow your search, first determine how much hold you want from the hairspray.

If the bottle says it offers "flexible" hold, it is one of the lightest formulas that will give you a bit of hold and shine, and is a good option for everyday looks. "Strong" hold is the next level, which will hold your hair in place if you occasionally have to face the elements like humidity or a bit of wind. "Maximum strength" is meant to hold your hair in place no matter how active you are, and are best for special occasions when you don't want your hair to move.

Other factors to consider are whether you want an aerosol hairspray that sprays continuously, or a pump hairspray that gives you short bursts of spray. You can also find non-sticky formulas and scent-free options and those that provide sun protection with SPF.

Look for hairsprays that are tailored to your hair type. Hairsprays for thin or fine hair will have specific ingredients that won't weigh hair down and will combat frizz and flyaways. When applying hairspray to fine hair, hold if further away from your head (about 12 inches away) so that you do not overload your hair.

If you have curly hair, look for a hairspray that is very lightweight and doesn't leave your hair feeling "crunchy." Instead, you still want to be able to run your fingers through your curls even after you apply hairspray.

Hairsprays that are infused with oils, like argan oil or macadamia oil, are best for dry hair types because they add an extra shine. You can also look for sprays that include ceramide, botanicals or other humidity-busting ingredients if your hair is damaged and tends to get frizzy as the weather changes. A good-quality hairspray is one of the quickest and easiest ways to get frizz and breakage under control.

Choosing the Right Combs and Brushes

Some people seem to think that brushes and combs are interchangeable styling tools. However, each one has a specific use – and there are many different types of each that are geared toward particular jobs and hair types. A comb should be used to detangle hair after you've washed it, and a brush is typically used on dry hair, but there are a few options to consider, depending on your hair's texture.

Combs

These plastic or metal styling tools are used for separating tangles and helping to create hairstyles. They come in various sizes and shapes and serve various purposes. An extra-wide tooth comb is essential for all hair types. Because there is so much space between the teeth, these are best for detangling or even for distributing conditioner throughout your hair while you're in the shower. The next comb, the wide-tooth comb, can be effective on either wet or dry hair to work through tangles without causing damage to any hair type.

A medium-tooth comb can help to style fine hair after it's been worked through with a wide-tooth or extra-wide-tooth comb. Teeth that are very close together are known as fine-tooth combs, found on tail, pin tail or cutting combs that are used for styling and trimming. A pin tail comb has a point on one end that can help you to separate your hair while you're styling it – either in rollers or flat ironing. You've likely seen your stylist working with a comb like this if you've ever had your hair colored or highlighted.

If you're using a comb on wet hair, be sure it is plastic, as a metal comb can damage fragile wet hair. Oily hair will benefit more from wider-tooth combs, but if you have dry hair, go for smaller-tooth combs that actually help the scalp to produce sebum.

Brushes

There may be nothing more confusing to purchase for your hair than your brush. They come in a variety of sizes and shapes and the bristles can be made of seemingly anything. The price of a brush varies from a few dollars to $50 or more. How do you know which one is right for your hair and worth the investment? You must know two things: which bristles are best for you and which shape will help you to achieve your desired style.

Nylon or plastic bristles are probably the most common and typically the least expensive. These synthetic bristles can be manufactured to be soft and flexible or very firm. If the bristles are close together and stiff, you'll have more control of how you style your hair. Brushes with metal bristles, on the other hand, should only be used on wigs because they can easily damage fine or aging hair.

Boar or porcupine bristles are more natural options that are gentler on the hair and help to smooth the cuticle layer of your hair. These types of bristles are very soft and flexible, so you may find them mixed in with nylon bristles on some brushes.

Brushes that are vented, meaning they do not have a solid surface, are best for blow drying the hair because the bristles are typically far apart and allow the air to flow through the brush, which speeds up the process. However, a vented brush won't add any styling benefits. A round brush, however, can help to create a bit of curl. Vented round brushes are the lightest weight and easy to use for longer periods of time without tiring out your hand and wrist – plus they dry your hair faster than a solid round brush center. A half-round brush is a more classic style that can help to create straighter styles when blow drying.

A brush that has a padding at the base of the bristles is great for brushing out long hair because the cushion is less resistant that hardbacked brushes, so the hair shouldn't stretch or break.

Styling Tools

Hair dryers

When choosing a hair dryer, you need to check out the wattage, heater and accessories.

To get the job done in a reasonable amount of time, look for one that is 1,750 watts or more. The thicker your hair, the higher the wattage should be – you can find some hair dryers with as much as 2,000 watts. A hair dryer with a ceramic heater is a good option if you are blow drying your hair straight. You'll also want an attachment that narrows the opening. However, if you have curly hair, purchase a diffuser, which delivers warm air to your hair without the blowing effect, which will cause curls to straighten.

Variable speed and heat options on your hair dryer are also a good options, so that you can adjust how much air and how warm it is. Remember, if it is so hot that it could burn your skin, it will also damage your hair.

Some women spend a lot of money to get their hair professionally blow dried. To get the sleek look yourself, start by applying styling serum to your damp hair. Use a wide- or extra-wide-tooth comb to evenly distribute it. Next, pin the majority of your hair on top of your head and start by blow drying a small portion of the bottom layer of your hair (at the nap of your neck). Use a large round brush to take up some of the hair at the roots. Direct the hair dryer from the roots to the end in a slow motion as you work the brush in the same direction.

If you want to create more volume at the roots, turn your head upside down and dry the roots first, using gravity to lift them up off your scalp. If you have short hair, a small round brush can continue to boost the volume of your hair.

Always angle the nozzle of the hairdryer pointing down so that it is moving in the same direction as the hair cuticle. Never aim the hair dryer up the hair shaft, as this will cause the cuticle to lift and look frizzy. Use the brush to angle any fringed hair around your face as you dry it. Finally, a cool-blast button can help to set the style. Finish with a shine serum or other finishing product that keeps frizz under control.

Curling irons

These come in a variety of sizes and materials that can be used for different styles and different hair types. They come with metal, ceramic or Teflon barrels at different price points. While they will all create curls, Teflon and ceramic barrels are best for eliminating frizz. If your hair is particularly prone to breakage, look for a curling iron that uses steam to heat it rather than dry heat, which can be more damaging.

Small barrel curling irons are best for fine or thin hair that respond quickly and easily to heated tools. Thick or coarse hair may need a curling iron that has adjustable heat and can be placed on a hotter setting. Care must be taken no matter what your hair type to ensure you are not keeping the curling iron in place for too long (no more than about 5 seconds).

Curling irons can be as small as 3/4 of an inch in diameter to 2 inches or larger. For a head full of voluminous, bouncing curls, you can alternate around your head with smaller and larger barrels to add more dimension and texture to your curled hair. Bigger barrels work best in the back of your head, while smaller barrels add definition near your face. When curling your hair, do not clamp the curler barrel around the ends of your hair. Instead, let them stick out a little bit as you wrap your hair around the barrel to avoid drying the ends further and causing split ends.

Flattening irons

Flat irons are relatively new to the hairstyling world as sleek, straight looks have become more popular. They come in a variety of materials and prices, but this is one tool that you don't want to skimp on. Opt for a flat iron that has ceramic plates and heats up from 140 degrees and 410 degrees (F). The lower heat works well on thin and fine hair, while the hotter settings are better for thick hair. If you're ready to invest, look for a ceramic flat iron that has tourmaline technology for super silky hair.

Before applying the flat iron to your hair, be sure to coat it with a thermal protection spray product that is formulated specifically for flat ironing your hair. When flat ironing, be sure to keep the iron in motion and don't stop and hold it on any section. Flat irons are very hot and can easily singe your hair. Follow with a shine serum or hairspray to hold its shape and tame fly-aways.

Hot rollers

These are another heated tool that you can use to make big, bouncy waves in your hair. They are typically sold in a kit where individual rollers are stored on metal rods that heat up. Once the plastic rollers are hot, you roll your dry hair (never use on wet hair) around them, secure them into place and wait until the cool down once again.

Some hot rollers have a spongy, velvety or Teflon coating around them, which is a good option if your hair is on the dry side. These will not snag as much in your hair and cause less damage. Ceramic-coated hot rollers are another good option because they do not have to heat up as much as plain plastic hot rollers. No matter which version you choose, be sure to start with a heat-protecting product on your hair, similar to what you would use when blow drying or flat ironing your hair.

If you want to get the same look without the damaging heat, try Velcro rollers. These come in a variety of sizes and can be rolled into place once your hair is about 80-90 percent dry. When rolling your hair into them, the Velcro conveniently grasps onto the hair to keep it rolled into place. If needed, give the rollers a little blast of heat to finish drying. When you unroll them, be careful not to tug on the Velcro, which can cause your hair to break.

Chapter 5: How to Grow Your Hair Longer

Long hair for women is a style that never goes out of fashion. It's a sign of sexy luxuriousness that men love and women try desperately to achieve. In fact, long hair has been such a traditional sign of femininity that women did not start to wear their hair cut short until after World War I. But even today, long hair, be it wavy, straight or curly, continues to be the pinnacle of womanly sensuality.

What is considered long hair? Your hair dresser will consider your hair to be "long" once it has grown past your clavicle bone. It may be all one length or cut into layers, but anything past that point puts you in the category.

Typically speaking, thicker, coarser hair can handle a longer cut better than fine, thin hair. But that doesn't have to be a fast-and-hard rule. If you can for your hair properly, any hair type can be grown out. One thing that actresses like Jennifer Aniston know about wearing long hair is that the cut is most important. Layering to best flatter your face shape is the key to getting your best, most-flattering look.

The Best Long Length for Your Hair

Curly hair

If you want to wear curly hair long, but have a round face, the key is to offset a round-shaped face by having the hair from the top of the head mostly straight, then start the curls at the mouth or below so that the curls do not make your round face look even wider. If you have all-over curly hair, be sure it hangs to your shoulders or lower, or else it will just make your entire face look fatter. Conversely, all-over curls look great on women with long-er faces because it visually adds width.

Wavy hair

If you have long, wavy hair it is probably on the thicker side, which is really the best of all worlds. You probably won't have to do much styling, but be sure your hairstylist cuts layers throughout to add some flowing texture. If you face is oval-shaped or long, have the layers start at your cheek or mouth to add some width the overall look. Women who have long faces and wear their hair flat and straight can tend to look like their faces are even longer than they are. Layers are a simple optical illusion to avoid that.

Straight hair

Flat-ironing your hair straight with a center part is a great way to add length to your face, making it a good option for women who have fuller faces. A side part can work as well for a sexier look. If you have a longer face, avoid stick-straight hair that hangs all one length. Add some layers starting at your cheeks or use a large-barrel curling iron to add some sexy texture.

Bangs and long hair

If you have long hair, no matter the texture, your best bet is to opt for a longer, side-swept bang. Short, blunt bangs that hang above your eyebrows tend to look odd with very long hair. If you do try bangs, ask you stylist to trim the sides of your hair at an angle for more texture that will look more sophisticated and complimentary to bangs. Also, be sure you have a substantial amount of bangs – not simply wispy fly-away-looking bangs. Bangs are a great way to shorten a face that has a long forehead. Be sure to have your hairstylist add some texture in your bangs with some mini-layers that will keep them from lying flat on your forehead.

Can you wear long hair at any age? The answer is yes. When you're in your 20s, you can try different styles and colors because you typically don't have to worry about wearing a more conservative cut. Plus, in your 20s, the cycle at which your hair grows is faster than when you get a bit older.

When you're in your 30s, you are probably juggling more than any other time – with small children, house maintenance and a career. If you'd still like the option to wear your hair long and sexy for a night out on the town, simply choose a cut that allows you to easily create a simple up-do or even a pony tail when you're in a hurry. Keep in mind that a pony tail can carry many different looks. High on your head will look more youthful, in the middle of your head looks sporty and low and the base of your neck is a more sophisticated style that looks polished enough to wear at work. Choose pony tail holders that match your hair color or wrap a bit of your own hair around the pony tail holder for a finished look.

In your 40s, don't feel like you have to chop your hair off. The best long-hair looks at this age are fuller, wavy layers. This adds vitality to a face that is beginning to show some signs of aging. Also, your hair might start to feel drier and may be more susceptible to breaking and split ends. Get regular (every six to eight weeks) haircuts and be sure to follow a good hair-care routine. Try adding some highlights and/or lowlights to keep the color looking interesting.

In your 50s and 60s, you may opt to keep some length, but a bit shorter – maybe around shoulder length. This is a universally flattering length and works well with hair that might be thinning a bit or has a drier texture. Accenting your natural texture here is a good option because doing too much styling with older hair will tend to look quite dated. Keep it soft and natural.

How to Grow Your Hair Longer

There may be times in your life when it seems that your hair is growing faster than other times. That's because for environmental or biological reasons, your hair growth cycle has sped up or slowed down. The cycle is broken down into three stages: 1. The growing phase for your hair can last between two and six years, depending on your genetic makeup. The vast majority of your hair follicles are in the growing stage. 2. When your hair starts to go through the natural cycle of falling out, it's in the shedding phase. If your hair is normal and healthy, new hair will grow where the old hair was. 3. Your hair naturally goes through a resting phase for a few weeks between the growing and shedding phases.

Your hair may reach its "terminal" length, which simply means it won't grow uniformly longer. It's best to stop at that length. Also, as you age, the growth cycle may slow down at the follicle level and each strand may even grow thinner. You can still wear it long, if looks healthy and you maintain it well.

Your hair will continue to go through this cycle unless you have a hair-loss issue, which, for women, is usually due to a medical or stress issue. If your hair is naturally cycling, be sure to keep it healthy with regular trims. Otherwise, you'll end up with split ends that look dry and unhealthy.

Because nutrition is key for beautiful hair, some experts believe that you can alter your diet and boost your hair's growing ability. For longer hair, be sure you are eating foods that contain folic acid, like soybeans and wheat; vitamin A, like spinach and milk, to keep your scalp healthy; vitamin B in foods like green vegetables and lean red meat, which is believed to prevent hair loss; and vitamin C, like citrus fruits, broccoli and berries, for healthier hair overall.

Maintaining long hair is essential. The diet described above will certainly help, as will cutting off any damaged hair, trimming a half an inch every eight weeks and using a deep conditioner or hair mask once a week to keep the ends moisturized and healthy. Also, keep in mind that because hair grows about a half an inch a month, any hair that is 10 inches long from the scalp is about two years old. That hair needs a lot of care and less damaging elements like excessive blow drying, flat ironing or curling. It can damage more easily, so be gentle with it and condition every time you wash it. Also, brush your hair starting with the bottom of your hair to gently detangle knots before running the brush through the full length of your hair.

Another Option: Extensions

It's no secret that celebrities like Kim Kardashian and Jessica Simpson rely on hair extensions to make their natural hair look thicker and longer. They are becoming more mainstream and easier to use in order to totally transform your look.

There are four major benefits to wearing hair extensions. 1. You can correct a bad haircut and extensions can be used to camouflage any problems while it grows back out. 2. Boost or experiment with your color with a complementary shade in the extensions. 3. You can also add volume to thin or thinning hair and create a sexier look. 4. Improve the texture of your hair with extensions that blend into your hair to make it wavier or curlier.

Hair extensions come in two types: human hair and synthetic hair. Both have their benefits and drawbacks. Human hair is more natural looking, but after it is washed several times it can lose its natural glossy look. It can be cut or colored into any style, but it's typically heavier and more expensive than synthetic hair. On the other hand, synthetic extensions is lighter weight and less expensive. However, it doesn't have the same natural bounce as real hair and doesn't blend as well with your natural hair. It also may not respond to coloring or styling as well, but it may be a good option if you want to test out what a long hairdo might look on you.

Temporary hair extensions are typically put in place with a comb that you can attach yourself. These are typically made of synthetic hair and a good option if you simply want longer hair for a short time, like a special occasion.

More permanent extensions are put into place with a weave. They are braided into a skirt that is stitched horizontally into your natural hair. Another method is called wefts, which are bonded into your hair – not your scalp – with an adhesive. These can last up to six months, but they must be inserted and removed by a hairstylist, and can cost up to $2,000. Plus, your extensions will require a fair amount of care. Be sure to consult with an experienced hairstylist to determine which style is best for you before committing to extensions.

Fact and Fiction about Growing Longer Hair

At some point in every woman's life, she'll want longer hair. There are lots of myths and misconceptions about what it takes to grow your hair longer. Here are some truths to know:

Trimming your hair won't make it grow faster. It is a common belief that if you trim your hair regularly that it will grow faster. The truth is that it will look better because you're eliminating any scraggly split ends. However, the growth of your hair is based on the growth cycle that begins within the hair follicles in your scalp. Trimming the ends doesn't do anything to alter the growth cycle. It simply makes your hair look better maintained. (And is highly recommended for long hair.)

Adding oil to your scalp will not help the growth cycle. Women of color have been sold on the fact that adding oil to the scalp will make their hair grow faster. Actually, it can clog your hair follicles and have the opposite effect. Instead, use the oil on the actual strands of your hair to help moisturize it and keep it looking shiny.

What you do, indeed, affect your hair growth. Your hair is a living element on your body, and as such needs good nutrition to perform optimally. Vitamins and supplements with vitamin A, B and C as well as folic acid, magnesium and beta-carotene will directly affect the health of your hair. In addition to those, practicing good-health habits will promote better hair growth as well. Be sure to drink lots of water to keep you hydrated from head-to-toe, eat lots of green vegetables and add more protein to your diet. Since your hair is also a protein, it needs this nutrient to look its best.

In addition, following a healthy lifestyle will make your hair – no matter the length – look better. Avoid smoking, which can cause your hair to go gray prematurely. In fact, research shows that smokers are four times more likely to have gray hair than people who do not smoke. If you're in the sun a lot, be sure to use sunscreen on your scalp or wear a hat. A sunburn – or excessive tanning – can actually lead to hair loss because it damages the hair follicle. Also, do not share your brushes or hairstyling tools with other people. These can harbor parasites that you can pick up if you use someone else's brush. In addition, be sure to keep your stress levels down by performing relaxing routines every day. Stress is one of the most common reasons women experience hair thinning or loss. Give yourself a daily head massage to get the blood circulating in the scalp – and it feels great and is relaxing, as well.

Avoiding chemicals will not make your hair grow faster. While certain chemicals used for curling, straightening and coloring your hair can dry the hair out or even damage it, it does nothing to alter the growth cycle.

Having longer hair doesn't cause it to grow more slowly, as some people believe. It may seem to slow down because you have developed split ends. These frayed ends can actually travel up the hair shaft, making it not only look shorter, but also frizzier and un- healthy. You can only remove split ends by cutting them off, but not by using any type of product. It's best to entirely cut the length of the split ends and start fresh. Try to get trims every six to eight weeks.

Men actually do prefer longer hair on women. In many studies and surveys, men overwhelmingly choose images of women with longer hair as more attractive than those with shorter hair.

Long-Hair Tips

Now that you know what won't work for growing your hair longer, keep these tips in mind for growing out your hair naturally and beautifully:

- Start fresh by cutting off all split ends

- Get small trims every six to eight weeks

- Ask for a hairstylist who is experienced in all aspects of working with long hair

- Lay off the heated hairstyling tools like the hair drier, flat iron and curling iron to give your hair a break from time to time. These often inspire split ends.

- Ease off chemicals like curling, straightening or coloring products. They do damage to your hair, so use them judiciously.

- If you wear buns, pony tails or braids, do so loosely. Tightly pulling on your hair can actually cause it to break or fall out.

- Use fabric-covered hair ties, not bare elastic, which can cause your hair to break.

- Be gentle with your hair at all times.

- Try sleeping on satin or silk pillowcases, which are less likely to snag on your hair, which can cause breakage.

- After washing, don't rub your hair in a towel, which can cause it to tangle. Instead, blot it gently.

Chapter 6: Change Your Hair

When it comes to our hair, it seems the grass is always straighter, curlier, darker or lighter and we're never 100 percent happy with what we've got naturally. That's why there's an entire industry built around providing services to change the color or texture of our hair or to reverse damage that has been done. While there are many professional options, there are also some ways to change your hair naturally, which is also included in this chapter.

Hair coloring

Women have always wanted to change the natural color of their hair. Over the decades, hair coloring treatments have diversified and you can now temporarily color your hair, color only a portion of it, go for a dramatic change or simply touch up grays. Coloring products have been known to be full of chemicals and can damage the hair (it is even rec-ommended that pregnant women stay away from hair coloring). However, during recent years less-damaging products have begun to surface on the market.

Some salons offer champagne rinses, which are said to add a glow to the hair and even lighten it a bit. (You can try this at home by spritzing champagne onto damp roots and combing it through before using a hair dryer). There are also many coloring products that are organic, herb-based formulas that do not contain ammonia and are just as effective as chemical-based coloring products. With repeated use, chemical coloring products will dry out the hair and make it brittle.

Few people can successfully go from one extreme to the other when coloring their hair. However, if you were a blonde when you were a child, but have grown up to have darker hair, your skin tone will likely support going lighter once again. If this is a drastic change and you have pretty dark roots, keep in mind that staying blonde will be an expensive endeavor. But you can add in some lighter highlights to your roots from time to time to hold off going back to the hairstylist for a while.

Going brunette can really resolve a lot of hair-related sins. Because brown hair reflects the light better than any other shade, it can look healthier and shiner than blonde. Warm tones will complement nearly any complexion, especially when paired with caramel highlights and darker low lights that add texture without having to cut layers into your hair.

Trying to go redder is even trickier. It's best for people who have fair skin and don't mind making a bold statement with their hair – especially if it is a drastic change from blonde or brown. Everyone will notice – there's no way around that fact. Red hair coloring will fade faster than any others, so try to keep your locks out of the sun, and don't over-shampoo your hair.

It's a good idea to use shampoo, conditioner and other hair-care products that are specifically designed for color-treated hair. Look for the ingredient eugenol, which will keep your color from fading. This not only locks in essential moisture, but can also stop colored hair from turning "brassy," which is a common complaint among people who color their hair. One way to combat brassiness in colored hair is to add some darker low lights to balance out the color and keep the hair protected from the sun, which can turn even non-colored hair brassy.

If you want to try other natural coloring treatments, look for a shampoo that includes chamomile, which can highlight light hair. Shampoos with henna can give darker hair a bit of red undertones without damaging chemicals.

Hair straightening

There are a plethora of options when it comes to straightening your hair. There are many chemicals that are used today, including lye relaxers, which are ideal for very kinky hair, texturizers used when blow drying and Japanese straightening treatments, which holds its new, straight texture until new hair grows out. The Brazilian Keratin Treatments, which were quite popular a few years ago, have been banned in many countries because the keratin is mixed with formaldehyde, which has been shown to cause skin irritations, nausea, nose bleeds and an increased risk of cancer.

If you have your hair chemically straightened, keep in mind that the chemicals will weaken your hair a bit, and you must take care to keep it in good condition. Limit the amount of heat you use and always use a wide-tooth comb to detangle your hair.

There are many over-the-counter products that will help to straighten your hair with the aid of a hair dryer and/or a flat iron. Be sure to use a protective product first so that your hair is protected from the heat. While these are temporary straighteners, you won't be exposed to the chemicals used in many professional straightening treatments.

You can also try spritzing your hair with milk 20 minutes before shampooing it. Simply place milk in a spray bottle and spray your hair with it and comb through. Leave on for 20 minutes before washing and conditioning your hair. Be sure to rinse well.

Shine treatments

Our hair typically loses its healthy shine when it is overloaded with product residue or when we are under a great deal of stress or not practicing healthy eating habits. Some salons will offer deep conditioning treatments that will leave your hair incredibly shiny. They often apply the product and then put you under a hair dryer, which locks in the product's shine-enhancing properties. Some hair coloring formulas include non-ammonia, peroxide-based gloss that not only improves the color, but also the shine of the hair.

The summer months are particularly hard on your hair's shine because things like exposure to the sun and chlorine found in pools can strip away the glossy outer layer of your hair. Wear a hat to protect your hair from the elements and look for products that include SPF protection.

Also, shampoo with sulfates is a key contributor to hair that's lost its luster. Look for labels that say "sulfate-free" or "organic." For dry hair, use a boar-bristle brush, which will help distribute hair's natural oils through the strands.

Scalp and damage treatments

When you experience split ends or breakage, it's best to ask your hairstylist for help, but if you're having issues with your scalp, seek out a doctor. If your scalp is excessively dry and flaky or very oily or if your hair is breaking off near the scalp, you may have an underlying problem that only medical intervention can reverse.

However, if you have normal hair damage caused by excessive coloring, straightening or other chemical interactions or if it is overburdened with produce residue, you may needs to see a stylist for a thorough and deep cleansing, followed by intense moisturizing and perhaps a significant trim. Many salons offer restorative treatments for hair that's been through a lot.

You can also try a clarifying shampoo at home followed by a super-hydrating hair mask that you can purchase at a drug store. However, if you don't see improvement, you may need professional help for lifeless locks.

Treatments for Thinning or Aging Hair

As we age, our hair tends to become more dull and limp as well as more coarse and dry. Not to mention the gray hairs. There are ways, however, to improve the look of aging hair. All aging hair can be helped by stimulating the hair at the follicle. While you are shampooing and conditioning, simply give your scalp a massage. This brings blood flow to the follicle and activates the growth cycle, which may have slowed down over time. Aging hair will also greatly benefit from extra conditioning as well as the right haircut and color.

Before coloring aging hair, use a clarifying shampoo to remove any residue, as this will hamper the color's ability to absorb in your hair. Plus, go a little bit lighter on the length of the hair and keep the roots just a shade darker so that the hair will appear brighter around your face.

Just because you are getting older doesn't mean you have to wear your hair short. In fact, shoulder-length hair can do a lot to camouflage fine lines and wrinkles around the outside edges of the face or on the forehead. Plus, a good cut looks chic at any age. Ask for graduated, angled layers around your face and/or long bangs that you can wear swept over to the side. These two elements will create an instantly more modern look.

When coloring your hair, stay away from drastic colors, like going way too blonde or jet black. These extremes will make you look instantly older. Instead, opt for colors that mix light and dark shades of your color and look brighter and warmer against your skin. Good options are medium browns and honey blondes. (A hairstylist can choose the appropriate shades.) These will better camouflage any grays that sprout up, as well. You should only require coloring every two to three months, but if you feel like you need it more often, ask for a non-ammonia glaze that has fewer chemicals and will add shine to your hair.

If your hair is thinning, your hairstylist can suggest cuts that disguise any thinning areas and flatter your face. Also, highlights placed in your hair can give the illusion of thicker-looking hair. There are many treatments for thinning hair, including prescription drugs and creams and hair restoration treatments. However, hair loss is usually caused by an internal issue (such as hormone fluctuations, medications, poor diet, depression, etc.) and should be checked out by a physician to determine its cause before you spend money on products that may not help.

Chapter 7: Get Shinier, Prettier, Healthier Hair

While there is no shortage of products that promise to boost shine, reduce dullness and plump up your hair's volume, there is another way to help your hair – from the inside. Changing some of your eating habits can profoundly affect the health and look of your hair. The main goal is to avoid foods that have no nutritional value and, instead, eat foods that are high in nutrients.

Better Food Choices for Your Hair

Because your hair is comprised on protein, it only makes sense to include high-quality protein foods to your diet. Soy protein is an extremely low-fat option that is believed to stimulate hair growth. Other ideal proteins include milk and poultry.

If you have dry hair, it may be lacking in vitamin A, which directly affects the hair growth cycle and leave your hair looking even drier. Good proteins that include high-quality omega-3 fatty acids are the way to go to get the protein boost, vitamin A and extra hydration. Tuna, salmon, walnuts and flaxseed are good options. Eating cold-water fish, especially sardines, is also believed to help maintain your color because the hair is being strengthened with these additions to your diet.

If you find that your hair is breaking, the fatty acids and vitamin E can help here, as well. You'll also want to increase your selenium intake and maybe your overall calorie count. If you've ever been dieting, you know that your hair often pays a price when you eat too little food. Try to add nutrition, caloric foods like nuts and whole grains to your diet.

If your protein levels are low, you may notice that your hair is looking a bit dull. This is because the cuticle layer – the outermost layer of each strand of hair – has lifted, which makes hair look lifeless or frizzy. Lean meats, poultry and fish are good options, as are dark leafy greens.

For oily hair types, you may want to cut back on spicy or hot foods because they can actually cause your body temperature to rise and the skin on your head to heat and release your hair's natural oil into each strand of hair. In addition, eating too much sugar and fat can lead to more oil production, and generally are unhealthy for your skin, scalp and hair. Foods that counteract excessive oil production on your scalp include complex carbohydrates (whole wheat and fresh fruits and vegetables), olive oil and sushi. Stay away from overly processed and foods that are fried in oil.

Poor nutrition can also cause your hair to thin prematurely. If you are lacking in iron intake, boost it back up with lean red meats, green leafy vegetables, orange fruits and veggies and soy. Stay away from salty foods, as well. In addition, smoking, drinking, and extreme stress have also been linked to thinning hair and should be avoided or used in extreme moderation. Silica is a mineral that is found in peppers, sprouts and potatoes that has been found to slow down hair loss.

Everyone, no matter what type of hair, needs to be drinking at least two liters of water every day to get balanced hydration to the hair. To get even more hydration, eat fruits and vegetables that are rich in water, like celery, melons, tomatoes and lettuce.

Flaky scalp or dandruff can be combated with whole grains, which also promote cell repair. Avocados are a great overall food for hair as well, since they are full of vitamins and healthy fats that boost hair's hydration. Citrus fruits – oranges, grapefruits, lemons and limes, can help increase sebum production for people with dry hair. Vitamin B is particularly helpful in protected aging hair by strengthening it as its foundation and improves the circulatory system, which is important for hair follicle health. Try adding more green veggies, beans, nuts, carrots and seafood.

Lifestyle Changes to Improve Your Hair

In addition to your food choices, the way you treat your hair will make a big difference in how it looks from day-to-day. Here are some habits that will help:

When you bind your hair into a ponytail or braid, do so lightly. A super-tight hairstyle can easily cause your hair to break. Also, if you like to wear your hair tied back while you sleep, use a very loose ponytail holder.

Keep your hair protected from the sun. It's the number one factor in making hair look dull and lifeless. You can find shampoos, conditioners, serums and hairsprays that all include SPF protection against the sun's harmful rays. You may have used the sun to lighten your hair when you were younger, but as you age, this practice simply strips your hair of nutrients and its glossy cuticle begins to lift away and look frizzy and unappealing. If you can't find an SPF product, wear a hat. A wide-brimmed hat will cover all of your hair and protect your face as well. The sun is the enemy of youthful skin and hair, so stay covered up.

As often as possible, don't use heat-based tools. Overuse of hair dryers, curling irons, hot rollers and flat irons will eventually damage your hair beyond repair. Instead, scrunch some curling gel into your locks and let them dry naturally. You may find that your hair has excellent natural volume and even end up with a style you like better than your usual blow-out.

A recent study found that women who go through a divorce have more problems with thinning hair than other women. Are they literally pulling their hair out, or is it due to stress? Scientists say that stress is the main culprit, but often women also yank on their hair when they are having a bad day or twirl it incessantly while they are concentrating or even day dreaming. It's wise to practice stress-relieving habits, such as yoga or meditating on a daily basis. If you have particularly dry hair, a good stress reliever is to massage your scalp with a few small drops of essential oil on your fingertips. This will help the circulation in your scalp, increase blood flow and stimulate sebum production all while providing a relaxing massage.

Healthy Hair Habits

Some women know what it takes to always have beautiful, healthy hair. Here's how they do it:

- Don't shampoo too often and don't use too much shampoo. Unless you have really oily hair, you may be able to get away with washing your hair just two or three times a week. Try sprinkling on and brushing out a little bit of baking soda to keep oil at bay.

- As mentioned earlier, getting regular trims won't make your hair grow faster, but it will make it look healthier.

Plus, you'll stop any split ends from traveling up the hair shaft and causing more irreversible damage along the way.

- We've all heard the advice about brushing your hair 100 strokes before you go to bed every night. But that's not a good idea for everyone. Be sure to brush properly for your hair type. If you have dry hair, brushing somewhat regularly (a few times a day) can help your scalp produce more natural oils. However, if your hair is already oily, you don't want to stimulate more oil production. If you're an oily-hair type, try to stick with combing your hair to remove tangles and leave the brushing to the times when you're styling your hair only.

- Alternate the products that you use. If a product doesn't seem to work well anymore, it's not because the product has changed, but because your hair may have some residue built up. Use a cleansing shampoo for a few days, then try a different brand all together. After a month, you can go back to your favorite.

Undo Past Damage

Everyone experiences damaged hair in their lifetime. One of the most common problems, brittle hair with split ends, is usually caused by two main issues: over-styling (with heat and chemicals) and harshly treating hair by brushing it incorrectly and tying it into tight ponytails. Luckily there are many ways to start to repair it. You can almost instantly make it look better by using a non-ammonia, glossy hair color that is darker than your current shade.

Also, look for products that add moisture to your hair and are filled with hair-boosting ingredients like soy or wheat protein and natural oils. If your hair is naturally oily, use these types of products only on the length of your hair and avoid applying them near or on your scalp.

Also, be sure to get trims more frequently, try to wait to get your hair colored again and avoid wearing super-straight styles that will only call attention to frayed edges.

Color that is looking dull and drab has had too much – too much styling and too many chemicals. Ease off of shampooing your hair to every few days and try to air dry your hair and wear it naturally from time to time. Be sure you're using products with SPF protection and ones that promote shine.

If your hair is all-over frizzy, it may be due to genetics or too much time under the blow dryer. Your porous, probably wavy or curly hair type is prone to get super frizzy, so be sure you are not shampooing too often and that you are using a super-hydrating conditioner. Argan oil would be a good option for before and/or after styling your hair to help you lock in moisture.

Frizzier hair looks better if it's a bit longer because the weight of the hair will help it to lie down, rather than a short cut that can just poof out to the sides. Going a little darker with the color may help as well and limiting the amount of heat you use every day will help, too.

For hair that is limp and oily, be sure you are using a shampoo and conditioners that are free of oils. Your scalp is already producing enough oil and you don't want to add more in your hair-care products. Also, silicone is typically a dry-hair ingredient and won't be much help to oily hair. Unlike dry hair, going lighter with oily hair is a good solution. The lightening solution tends to make hair lighter, rather than weighted down against your scalp.

Conclusion

So now take a good, long look at your hair and determine what you'd like to do with it next. It's never too late to make a style change that can lift your spirits and drastically improve the look and health of your hair. For women, our hair is an extension of our personalities, and as your life changes through the years, don't be afraid to alter your hair. Keeping the same hairstyle for 10 or 20 years will only age you over time. Why not cut several inches off, try some highlights or straighten it from time to time?

And keep in mind you do not have to spend a fortune to have great-looking hair. A lot of the ingredients you need for cleansers, conditioners, masks and rinses can be found right in your kitchen. These natural alternatives will save you from drying and strip chemical-laden products that may look good in the short term, but can cause a lot of damage with repeated use.

That being said, keep in mind that a hairstylist is a professional who understands how hair grows and how it reacts to certain climates and products and can guide you to a hair routine, cut and style that's best for you and your lifestyle.

No matter what you put on the outside of your hair – whether it be to clean it, alter it or repair it – remember that you can improve all of those efforts by caring for your hair from the inside out, and now you have all the tools you need to achieve your healthiest strands ever.

Our hair is one of the first things people notice about us and judge about us. Keep yourself healthy and you'll be rewarded with shiny, glowing locks no matter what style you wear them in.